MEDITERRANEAN DIET COOKBOOK
FOR BEGINNERS

14 DAYS MEAL PLANS
&
50 HEALTHY RECIPES
TO GET YOU STARTED

WITH PICTURES

By Margaret Ralls

Mira Star Publisher web site:
www.mirastarpublisher.com

—

2

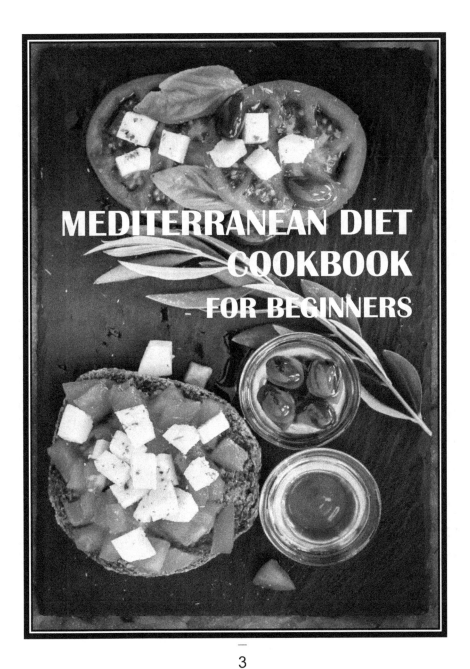

MEDITERRANEAN DIET
COOKBOOK
FOR BEGINNERS

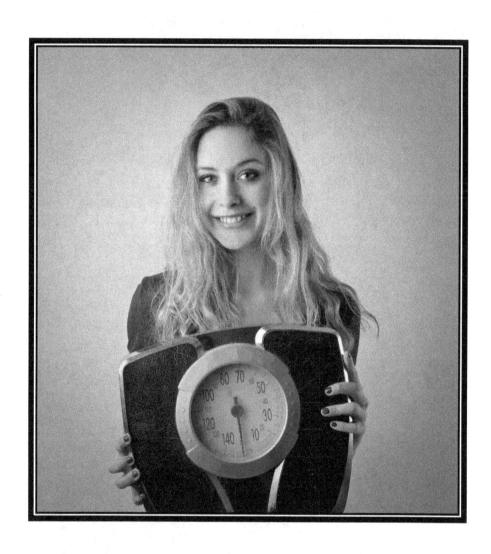

Contents

INTRODUCTION

The Mediterranean diet is a traditional diet that has roots that go back centuries. Indeed, the principles of this diet go back through time, well into the ancient past. People may have been eating this way from the very early days of agriculture thousands of years ago. Of course, they didn't have the insights that we do into the nature of human health. They didn't know about cholesterol, and many didn't live long enough to even develop heart disease, much less die from it. Simply getting enough food to eat was a challenge, and everyone was physically active because manual labor was necessary for survival. The diet developed as a result of the natural environment that existed around the Mediterranean region. The weather is perfect for growing olives and grapes, and the seas are rich in fatty fish. It was only natural that olive oil and red wine would become integral parts of the lifestyle of people and cultures living in this region.

Some also argue that the diet was consumed in the 1940s and 1950s simply as a result of the Second World War, which made processed food and meats harder to come by. There is some truth to this argument, but that is not a valid reason to avoid looking at the diet for its impact.

The reality is that the Mediterranean diet is timely; it is not out of date. At the present time, most people are suffering from health problems that are directly related to those that the Mediterranean diet solves. People are consuming large amounts of unhealthy, processed food. They often eat fast food that contains lots of sugars and corn syrup, along with unhealthy meat products. People are drinking sugary drinks and not getting the required amounts of fruits and vegetables. Many people never or rarely eat fatty fish.

Don't follow the old rule that you should only shop the perimeter of the grocery store. Today's supermarkets have Mediterranean Diet staples in every aisle—including the middle ones. While shopping, picture the Mediterranean Diet Pyramid inside your shopping cart: Half your cart should be fruits, vegetables, and plant-based foods, then fill up the rest with seafood, and so on.

Fresh produce section: What's in season? Seasonal fruits and vegetables are usually less expensive. Don't forget fresh herbs: Parsley, cilantro, basil, and mint can be budget-friendly ways to eat more always-in-season greens.

Fish counter: Ask questions. The fishmonger behind the counter is happy to steer you to inexpensive choices; he or she can also be a great source for recipes and cooking tips.

Canned fish aisle: There are lots of new additions here, including packets of tuna and salmon that are ready to eat with a fork. Most of the choices are simple and sustainable. Just pick your favorite or try something new, like sardines.

Frozen food aisle: The frozen food aisle is an ideal place to finish filling your cart with fruit and veggies. In general, frozen fruits and vegetables are just as nutritious as fresh, as they are frozen at the peak of freshness. Choose any vegetable without sauce. We buy frozen fruits to go into every breakfast, from cereal to yogurt. Frozen fish fillets are healthy, convenient choices, and because they're often frozen individually, you can cook just what you need.

Rice and grains aisle: In general, you'll find most whole grains here, in the natural food's aisle, or in the bulk food section. To make sure the grains are whole, search for these words on the Nutrition Facts label: oats, bulgur, wheat berries, rye berries, or whole [name of grain], such as whole wheat. Look for faro, bulgur, quinoa, sorghum, spelt, barley, brown rice (instant and regular), and wild rice without any added flavors or seasonings.

Bulk food section: This area, with foods in open bins, makes food shopping fun. Here's where you can buy small amounts of things to taste, without spending a lot on full packages of whole grains, beans, and dried fruits.

Dairy case: From low-fat to full fat, we promote eating the type of milk, cheese, or yogurt that you prefer. Products with more fat will have more calories, but we find that they are more filling and flavorful, and often you can use less in a recipe. When it comes to yogurt, we prefer plain, but if you are buying flavored yogurt, compare the amount of added sugar to other flavored yogurts and go with the lowest number. (The total sugar amount on the label also includes the lactose and fructose—those naturally occurring sugars found in dairy and fruit.) Or better yet, buy the plain and add your own fruit.

The Mediterranean diet does not specify a number of calories to be ingested in order to achieve weight loss, but contributes to a healthy lifestyle by eating healthy, wholesome foods that allow our body to gain an appropriate weight over time. It is possible to follow the Mediterranean diet every day and share this style of well-being with the whole family.

However, in order to lose weight, a low-calorie diet is necessary.

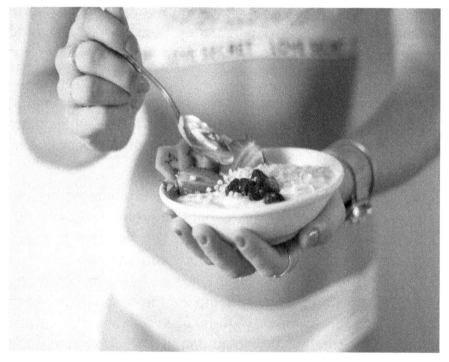

A daily calorie intake of between 1200 and 1500 will certainly allow you to lose up to 2 pounds per week. Clearly this is a regime that cannot be followed for a long time as it is very restricted.

Below you will find 14 days of meal plans:

- **14 BREAKFAST RECIPES**
- **14 LUNCH RECIPES**
- **14 DINNER RECIPES**
- **+8 DESSERTS**

The meal with the highest number of calories and an intake of cereals and fruit should be eaten in the morning to allow the body to have the sugars and strength to face the day.

Lunch should be a quick and light meal, because it allows us to stay alert and active after lunch and continue our activities at work without falling into the drowsiness that comes from eating a heavy, high-calorie meal.

In the evening it would be better to eat meals with a higher protein content such as fish, white meat, eggs.

For dessert lovers, there are 8 recipes from the Mediterranean diet that will give you the right energy when your strength wanes. It's up to you to decide when to eat them, we always recommend before 2pm to allow the body to work off the calories.

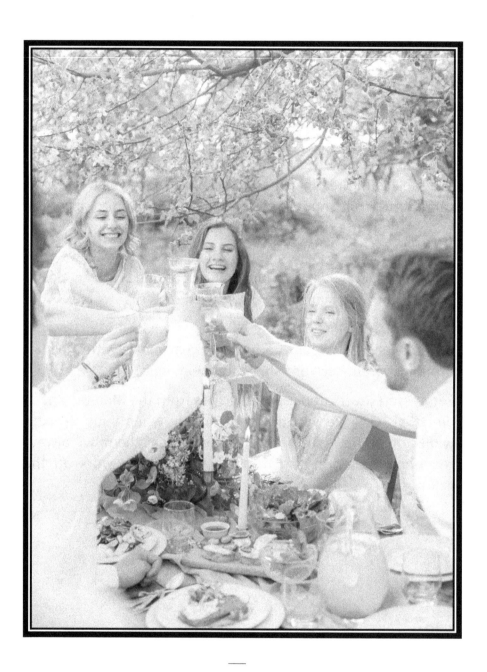

Chapter 1

14 DAYS - BREAKFAST

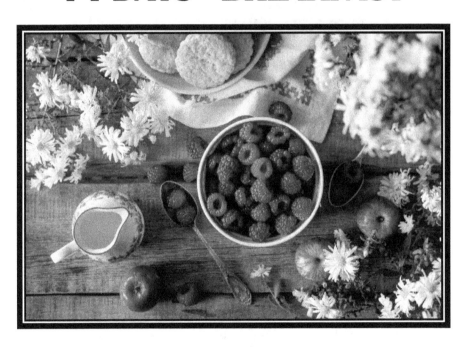

DAY 01

Avocado Chickpea Pizza

Preparation time: 20 minutes
Cooking Time: 20 minutes
Servings: 2

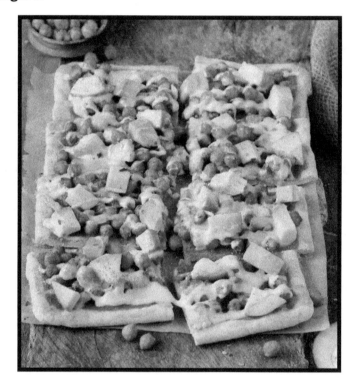

NUTRITION
Calories 416, Fiber 24.5, Protein 15.4g, Carbs: 36.6g, Fat: 24.5g

INGREDIENTS

- **1** AND ¼ CUPS CHICKPEA FLOUR
- **A** PINCH OF SALT AND BLACK PEPPER
- **1** AND ¼ CUPS WATER
- **2** TABLESPOONS OLIVE OIL
- **1** TEASPOON ONION POWDER
- **1** TEASPOON GARLIC, MINCED
- **1** TOMATO, SLICED
- **1** AVOCADO, PEELED, PITTED AND SLICED
- **2** OUNCES GOUDA, SLICED
- **¼** CUP TOMATO SAUCE
- **2** TABLESPOONS GREEN ONIONS, CHOPPED

DIRECTION

1. In a bowl, mix the chickpea flour with salt, pepper, water, the oil, onion powder and the garlic, stir well until you obtain a dough, knead a bit, put in a bowl, cover and leave aside for 20 minutes.
2. Transfer the dough to a working surface, shape a bit circle, transfer it to a baking sheet lined with parchment paper and bake at 425 degrees F for 10 minutes.
3. Spread the tomato sauce over the pizza, also spread the rest of the ingredients and bake at 400 degrees F for 10 minutes more.
4. Cut and serve for breakfast.

DAY 02

BAKED OMELET MIX

Preparation time: 45 minutes
Cooking Time: 12 minutes
Servings: 12

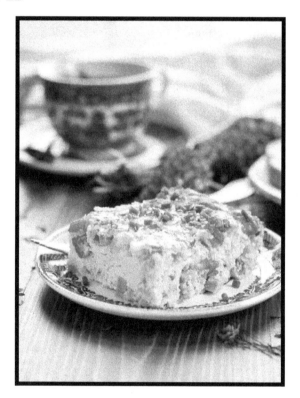

NUTRITION
Calories 186, Protein 10g, Carbs: 5g, Fat: 13g, Fiber 1g

Ingredients

- **12** EGGS, WHISKED
- **8** OUNCES SPINACH, CHOPPED
- **2** CUPS ALMOND MILK
- **12** OUNCES CANNED ARTICHOKES, CHOPPED
- **2** GARLIC CLOVES, MINCED
- **5** OUNCES FETA CHEESE, CRUMBLED
- **1** TABLESPOON DILL, CHOPPED
- **1** TEASPOON OREGANO, DRIED
- **1** TEASPOON LEMON PEPPER
- **A** PINCH OF SALT
- **4** TEASPOONS OLIVE OIL

Direction

1. Heat up a pan with the oil over medium-high heat, add the garlic and the spinach and sauté for 3 minutes.
2. In a baking dish, combine the eggs with the artichokes and the rest of the ingredients.
3. Add the spinach mix as well, toss a bit, bake the mix at 375 degrees F for 40 minutes, divide between plates and serve for breakfast.

DAY 03

STUFFED SWEET POTATOES

Cooking Time: 40 minutes
Servings: 8

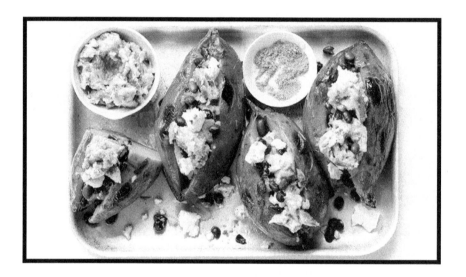

NUTRITION
Calories 308, Fat 2 g, Carbohydrate 38 g, Fiber 8g, Protein 7g

INGREDIENTS

- **8** SWEET POTATOES, PIERCED WITH A FORK
- **14** OUNCES CANNED CHICKPEAS, DRAINED AND RINSED
- **1** SMALL RED BELL PEPPER, CHOPPED

- **1** TABLESPOON LEMON ZEST, GRATED
- **2** TABLESPOONS LEMON JUICE
- **3** TABLESPOONS OLIVE OIL
- **1** TEASPOON GARLIC, MINCED
- **1** TABLESPOON OREGANO, CHOPPED
- **2** TABLESPOONS PARSLEY, CHOPPED
- **A** PINCH OF SALT AND BLACK PEPPER
- **1** AVOCADO, PEELED, PITTED AND MASHED
- ¼ CUP WATER
- ¼ CUP TAHINI PASTE

DIRECTION

1. Arrange the potatoes on a baking sheet lined with parchment paper, bake them at 400 degrees F for 40 minutes, cool them down and cut a slit down the middle in each.
2. In a bowl, combine the chickpeas with the bell pepper, lemon zest, half of the lemon juice, half of the oil, half of the garlic, oregano, half of the parsley, salt and pepper, toss and stuff the potatoes with this mix.
3. In another bowl, mix the avocado with the water, tahini, the rest of the lemon juice, oil, garlic and parsley, whisk well and spread over the potatoes.
4. Serve cold for breakfast.

DAY 04

CAULIFLOWER FRITTERS

Preparation time: 50 minutes
Servings: 4

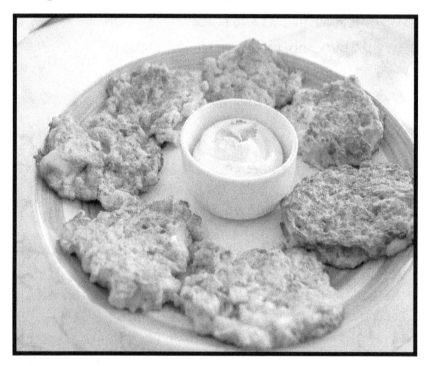

NUTRITION
Calories 333 Fat 12.6 g, Carbohydrate 44.7 g Fiber 12.8 g, Protein
13.6 g

INGREDIENTS

- **30** OUNCES CANNED CHICKPEAS, DRAINED AND RINSED
- **2 AND ½** TABLESPOONS OLIVE OIL
- **1** SMALL YELLOW ONION, CHOPPED
- **2** CUPS CAULIFLOWER FLORETS CHOPPED
- **2** TABLESPOONS GARLIC, MINCED
- **A** PINCH OF SALT AND BLACK PEPPER

DIRECTION

1. Spread half of the chickpeas on a baking sheet lined with parchment pepper, add 1 tablespoon oil, season with salt and pepper, toss and bake at 400 degrees F for 30 minutes.
2. Transfer the chickpeas to a food processor, pulse well and put the mix into a bowl.
3. Heat up a pan with the ½ tablespoon oil over medium-high heat, add the garlic and the onion and sauté for 3 minutes.
4. Add the cauliflower, cook for 6 minutes more, transfer this to a blender, add the rest of the chickpeas, pulse, pour over the crispy chickpeas mix from the bowl, stir and shape medium fritters out of this mix.
5. Heat up a pan with the rest of the oil over medium-high heat, add the fritters, cook them for 3 minutes on each side and serve for breakfast.

DAY 05

TUNA SALAD

Preparation time: 24 minutes
Cooking time: 60 minutes
Servings: 4

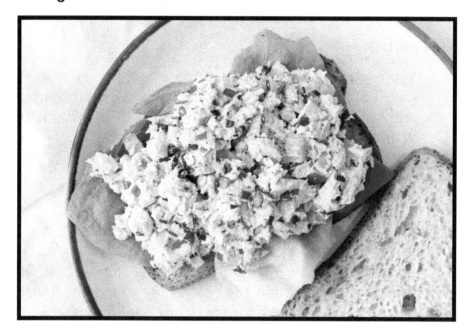

NUTRITION

Calories 250, Fat 17.3 g, Fiber 0.8, Carbohydrate 2.7 g, Protein 10.1 g

INGREDIENTS

- **12** OUNCES CANNED TUNA IN WATER, DRAINED AND FLAKED
- **¼** CUP ROASTED RED PEPPERS, CHOPPED
- **2** TABLESPOONS CAPERS, DRAINED
- **8** KALAMATA OLIVES, PITTED AND SLICED
- **2** TABLESPOONS OLIVE OIL
- **1** TABLESPOON PARSLEY, CHOPPED
- **1** TABLESPOON LEMON JUICE
- **A** PINCH OF SALT AND BLACK PEPPER

DIRECTION

1. In a bowl, combine the tuna with roasted peppers and the rest of the ingredients, toss, divide between plates and serve for breakfast.

DAY 06
LEEKS AND EGGS MUFFIN

Preparation time: 10 minutes
Cooking time: 5 minutes
Servings: 4

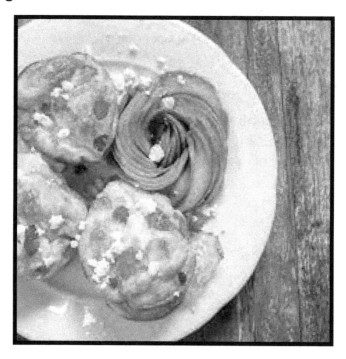

NUTRITION
Calories 308, Fat 19.4g, Fiber 1.7, Carbohydrate 8.7 g, Protein
24.4 g

INGREDIENTS

- 3 EGGS, WHISKED
- ¼ CUP BABY SPINACH
- 2 TABLESPOONS LEEKS, CHOPPED
- 4 TABLESPOONS PARMESAN, GRATED
- 2 TABLESPOONS ALMOND MILK
- COOKING SPRAY
- 1 SMALL RED BELL PEPPER, CHOPPED
- SALT AND BLACK PEPPER TO THE TASTE
- 1 TOMATO, CUBED
- 2 TABLESPOONS CHEDDAR CHEESE, GRATED

DIRECTION

1. In a bowl, combine the eggs with the milk, salt, pepper and the rest of the ingredients except the cooking spray and whisk well.
2. Grease a muffin tin with the cooking spray and divide the eggs mixture in each muffin mould.
3. Bake at 380 degrees F for 20 minutes and serve them for breakfast.

DAY 07

VEGGIE QUICHE

Preparation Time: 6 minutes
Cooking Time: 55 minutes
Servings: 8

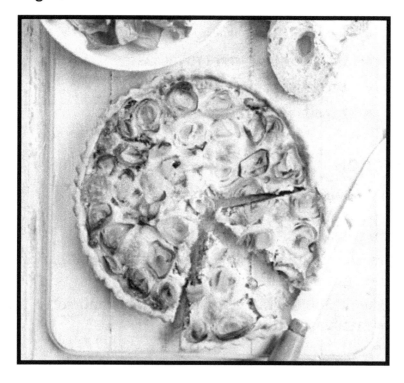

NUTRITION

Calories: 211 kcal, Carbs: 12.5g, Fat: 14.4g, Protein: 8.6g. Fiber 1.4

INGREDIENTS

- ½ CUP SUN-DRIED TOMATOES, CHOPPED
- 1 PREPARED PIE CRUST
- 2 TABLESPOONS AVOCADO OIL
- 1 YELLOW ONION, CHOPPED
- 2 GARLIC CLOVES, MINCED
- 2 CUPS SPINACH, CHOPPED
- 1 RED BELL PEPPER, CHOPPED
- ¼ CUP KALAMATA OLIVES, PITTED AND SLICED
- 1 TEASPOON PARSLEY FLAKES
- 1 TEASPOON OREGANO, DRIED
- 1/3 CUP FETA CHEESE, CRUMBLED
- 4 EGGS, WHISKED
- 1 AND ½ CUPS ALMOND MILK
- 1 CUP CHEDDAR CHEESE, SHREDDED
- SALT AND BLACK PEPPER TO THE TASTE

DIRECTION

1. Heat up a pan with the oil over medium-high heat, add the garlic and onion and sauté for 3 minutes.

2. Add the bell pepper and sauté for 3 minutes more.

3. Add the olives, parsley, spinach, oregano, salt and pepper and cook everything for 5 minutes.

4. Add tomatoes and the cheese, toss and take off the heat.

5. Arrange the pie crust in a pie plate, pour the spinach and tomatoes mix inside and spread.

6. In a bowl, mix the eggs with salt, pepper, the milk and half of the cheese, whisk and pour over the mixture in the pie crust.

7. Sprinkle the remaining cheese on top and bake at 375 degrees F for 40 minutes.

8. Cool the Quiche down, slice and serve for breakfast.

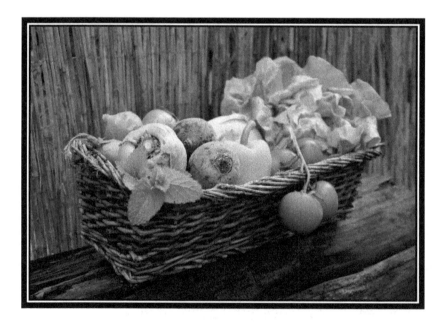

DAY 08

GARBANZO BEAN SALAD

Preparation Time: 5 minutes
Servings: 4

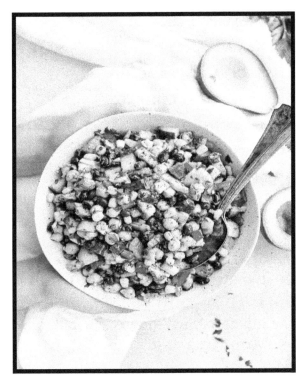

NUTRITION
Calories: 268kcal, Carbs: 21.8g, Fat: 16g, Fiber 7g, Protein: 9g,
Fiber 55.4

INGREDIENTS

- **1** AND **½** CUPS CUCUMBER, CUBED
- **15** OUNCES CANNED GARBANZO BEANS, DRAINED AND RINSED
- **3** OUNCES BLACK OLIVES, PITTED AND SLICED
- **1** TOMATO, CHOPPED
- **¼** CUP RED ONION, CHOPPED
- **5** CUPS SALAD GREENS
- **A** PINCH OF SALT AND BLACK PEPPER
- **½** CUP FETA CHEESE, CRUMBLED
- **3** TABLESPOONS OLIVE OIL
- **1** TABLESPOON LEMON JUICE
- **¼** CUP PARSLEY, CHOPPED

DIRECTION

1. In a salad bowl, combine the garbanzo beans with the cucumber, tomato and the rest of the ingredients except the cheese and toss.
2. Divide the mix into small bowls, sprinkle the cheese on top and serve for breakfast.

DAY 09

QUINOA AND EGGS SALAD

Preparation Time: 5 minutes
Servings: 4

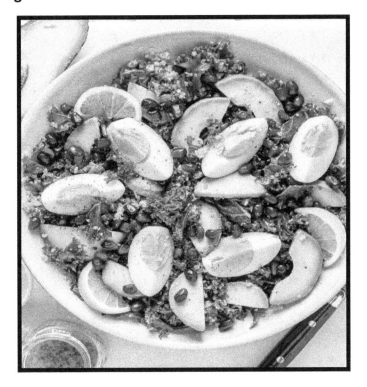

NUTRITION
Calories 519, Fat 32.4, Fiber 11, Carbs 43.3, Protein 19.1

INGREDIENTS

- **4** EGGS, SOFT BOILED, PEELED AND CUT INTO WEDGES
- **2** CUPS BABY ARUGULA
- **2** CUPS CHERRY TOMATOES, HALVED
- **1** CUCUMBER, SLICED
- **1** CUP QUINOA, COOKED
- **1** CUP ALMONDS, CHOPPED
- **1** AVOCADO, PEELED, PITTED AND SLICED
- **1** TABLESPOON OLIVE OIL
- **½** CUP MIXED DILL AND MINT, CHOPPED
- **A** PINCH OF SALT AND BLACK PEPPER JUICE OF **1** LEMON

DIRECTION

1. In a large salad bowl, combine the eggs with the arugula and the rest of the ingredients, toss, divide between plates and serve for breakfast.

DAY 10
ZUCCHINI AND QUINOA PAN

Preparation Time: 20 minutes
Servings: 4

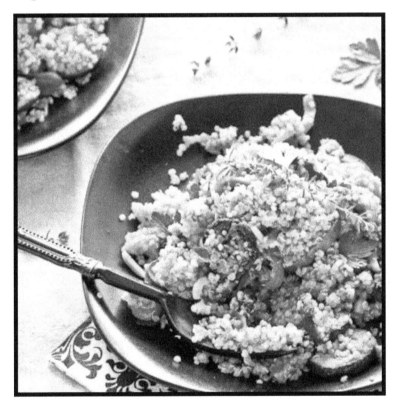

NUTRITION
Calories 310, Fat 11, Fiber 6, Carbs 42, Protein 11

INGREDIENTS

- **1** TABLESPOON OLIVE OIL
- **2** GARLIC CLOVES, MINCED
- **1** CUP qUINOA
- **1** ZUCCHINI, ROUGHLY CUBED
- **2** TABLESPOONS BASIL, CHOPPED
- **¼** CUP GREEN OLIVES, PITTED AND CHOPPED
- **1** TOMATO, CUBED
- **½** CUP FETA CHEESE, CRUMBLED
- **2** CUPS WATER
- **1** CUP CANNED GARBANZO BEANS, DRAINED AND RINSED **A** PINCH OF SALT AND BLACK PEPPER

DIRECTION

1. Heat up a pan with the oil over medium-high heat, add the garlic and quinoa and brown for 3 minutes.
2. Add the water, zucchinis, salt and pepper, toss, bring to a simmer and cook for 15 minutes.
3. Add the rest of the ingredients, toss, divide everything between plates and serve for breakfast.

DAY 11

ORZO AND VEGGIE BOWLS

Preparation Time: 5 minutes
Servings: 4

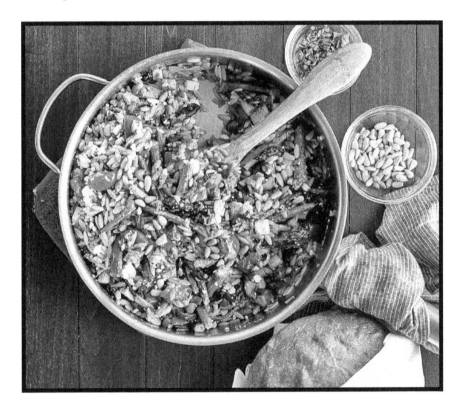

NUTRITION
Calories 411, Fat 17, Carbs 51, Protein 14, Fiber 13

INGREDIENTS

- **2 AND ½** CUPS WHOLE-WHEAT ORZO, COOKED
- **14** OUNCES CANNED CANNELLINI BEANS, DRAINED AND RINSED
- **1** YELLOW BELL PEPPER, CUBED
- **1** GREEN BELL PEPPER, CUBED
- **A** PINCH OF SALT AND BLACK PEPPER
- **3** TOMATOES, CUBED
- **1** RED ONION, CHOPPED
- **1** CUP MINT, CHOPPED
- **2** CUPS FETA CHEESE, CRUMBLED
- **2** TABLESPOONS OLIVE OIL
- **¼** CUP LEMON JUICE
- **1** TABLESPOON LEMON ZEST, GRATED
- **1** CUCUMBER, CUBED
- **1 AND ¼** CUP KALAMATA OLIVES, PITTED AND SLICED
- **3** GARLIC CLOVES, MINCED

DIRECTION

1. In a salad bowl, combine the orzo with the beans, bell peppers and the rest of the ingredients, toss, divide the mix between plates and serve for breakfast.

DAY 12
TAHINI PINE NUTS TOAST

Cooking Time: 5 minutes
Servings: 2

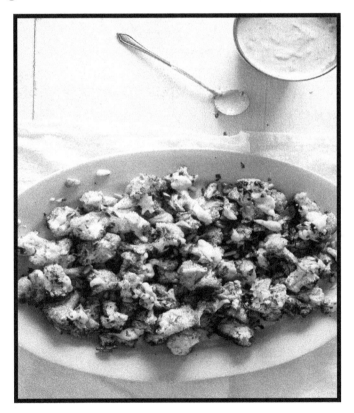

NUTRITION
Calories 142, Fat 7.6, Fiber 2.7, Carbs 13.7, Protein 5.8

37

INGREDIENTS

- **2** WHOLE WHEAT BREAD SLICES, TOASTED
- **1** TEASPOON WATER
- **1** TABLESPOON TAHINI PASTE
- **2** TEASPOONS FETA CHEESE, CRUMBLED
- JUICE OF ½ LEMON
- **2** TEASPOONS PINE NUTS
- **A** PINCH OF BLACK PEPPER

DIRECTION

1. In a bowl, mix the tahini with the water and the lemon juice, whisk really well and spread over the toasted bread slices.
2. Top each serving with the remaining ingredients and serve for breakfast.

DAY 13

CHEESY OLIVES BREAD

Preparation Time: 1h 40 minutes
Cooking Time: 30 minutes
Servings: 10

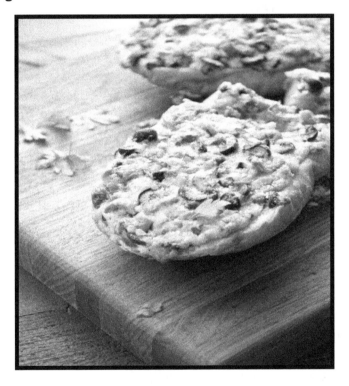

NUTRITION
Calories 251, Fat 7.3, Fiber 2.1, Carbs 39.7, Protein 6.7

INGREDIENTS

- **4 CUPS WHOLE-WHEAT FLOUR**
- **3 TABLESPOONS OREGANO, CHOPPED**
- **2 TEASPOONS DRY YEAST**
- **¼ CUP OLIVE OIL**
- **1 AND ½ CUPS BLACK OLIVES, PITTED AND SLICED**
- **1 CUP WATER**
- **½ CUP FETA CHEESE, CRUMBLED**

DIRECTION

1. In a bowl, mix the flour with the water, the yeast and the oil, stir and knead your dough very well.
2. Put the dough in a bowl, cover with plastic wrap and keep in a warm place for 1 hour.
3. Divide the dough into 2 bowls and stretch each ball really well.
4. Add the rest of the ingredients on each ball and tuck them inside well kneading the dough again.
5. Flatten the balls a bit and leave them aside for 40 minutes more.
6. Transfer the balls to a baking sheet lined with parchment paper and make a small slit in each and bake at 425 degrees F for 30 minutes.
7. Serve the bread as a Mediterranean breakfast.

DAY 14

RASPBERRIES AND YOGURT SMOOTHIE

Preparation Time: 5 minutes
Serving: 2

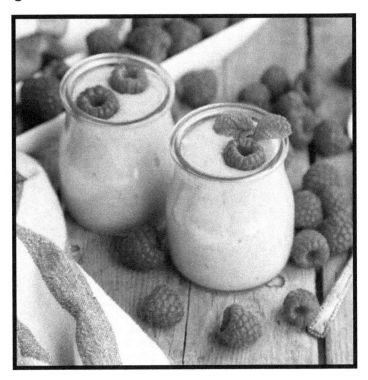

NUTRITION
Calories 245, Fat 9.5, Fiber 2.3, Carbs 5.6, Protein 1.6

INGREDIENTS

- **2** CUPS RASPBERRIES
- ½ CUP **GREEK** YOGURT
- ½ CUP ALMOND MILK
- ½ TEASPOON VANILLA EXTRACT

DIRECTION

1. In your blender, combine the raspberries with the milk, vanilla and the yogurt, pulse well, divide into 2 glasses and serve for breakfast.

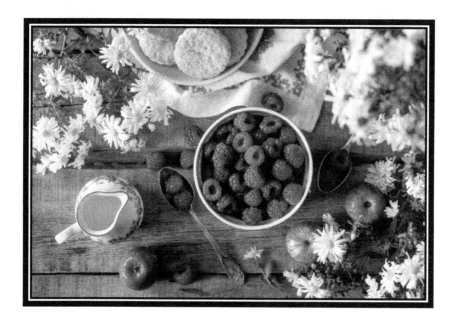

Chapter 2
14 DAYS - LUNCH

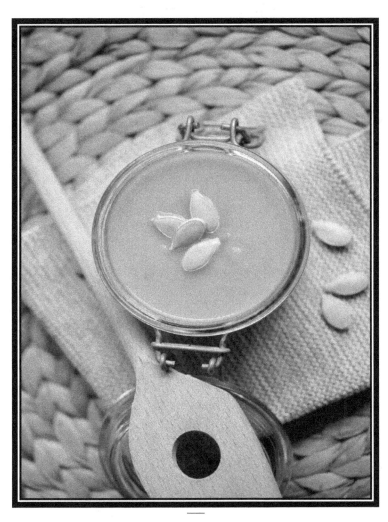

DAY 1

LINGUINE DREDGED IN TOMATO CLAM SAUCE

Preparation time: 10 minutes
Cooking Time: 10 minutes
Serving: 4

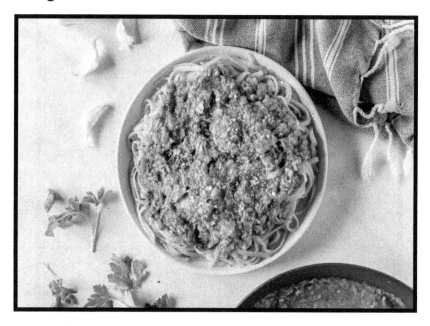

NUTRITION
Calories 394, Fat 5, Carbs 66, Protein 23

INGREDIENTS

- **1-POUND LINGUINE**
- **SALT AND BLACK PEPPER AS NEEDED**
- **1 TEASPOON EXTRA VIRGIN OLIVE OIL**
- **1 TABLESPOON GARLIC, MINCED**
- **1 TEASPOON FRESH THYME, CHOPPED**
- **½ TEASPOON RED PEPPER FLAKES**
- **1 CAN (15 OUNCES) SODIUM-FREE TOMATOES, DICED AND DRAINED**
- **1 CAN (15 OUNCE) CAN WHOLE BABY CLAMS, WITH JUICE**

DIRECTION

1. Cook the linguine accordingly.
2. While linguine cooks, heat olive oil in a large skillet over medium heat.
3. Add garlic, thyme, red pepper flakes and sauté for 3 minutes.
4. Stir in tomatoes and clams.
5. Bring sauce to boil and lower heat to low.
6. Simmer for 5 minutes.
7. Season with salt and pepper.
8. Drain cooked pasta and toss with sauce.
9. Garnish with parsley and serve.
10. *Enjoy!*

DAY 2

FAVORITE PEPPER SOUP

Preparation Time: 5 minutes
Cooking Time: 30 minutes
Serving: 6

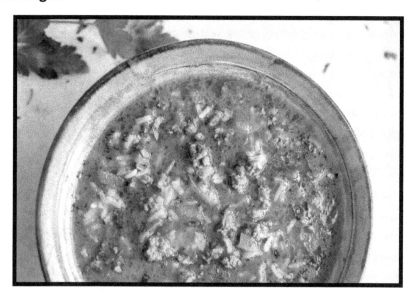

NUTRITION
Calories 162, Fat 3, Carbs 12, Protein 21

INGREDIENTS

- **1**-POUND LEAN GROUND BEEF
- **1** ONION, CHOPPED

- **1** LARGE GREEN PEPPER, CHOPPED
- **2** GARLIC CLOVES, MINCED
- **1** LARGE TOMATO, CHOPPED
- **2** TABLESPOONS TOMATO PASTE
- **2** TABLESPOONS ALL-PURPOSE FLOUR
- **¼** CUP UNCOOKED RICE
- **2** TABLESPOONS FRESH PARSLEY, CHOPPED
- **4** CUPS BEEF BROTH
- **2** TABLESPOONS OLIVE OIL SALT AND PEPPER AS NEEDED

DIRECTION

1. Take a large-sized pot and place it over medium heat.
2. Add oil and allow the oil to heat up.
3. Add flour and keep whisking until you have a thick paste.
4. Keep whisking for 3-4 minutes more while it bubbles and begins to thin.
5. Add chopped onion and sauté for 3-4 minutes.
6. Stir in tomato paste and beef.
7. Take a wooden spoon and stir to break the ground beef.
8. Cook for 5 minutes.
9. Add garlic, pepper and chopped tomatoes.
10. Mix well and combine.
11. Add broth and bring the mix to a light boil, reduce the heat to low and simmer for 30 minutes.

DAY 3

MUSHROOM AND BEEF RISOTTO

Preparation Time: 5 minutes
Cooking Time: 10 minutes
Serving: 4

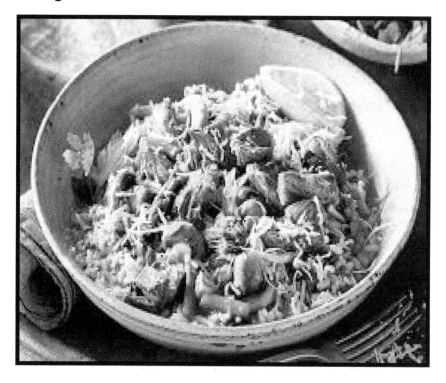

NUTRITION
Calories 378, Fat 12, Carbs 41, Protein 23

INGREDIENTS

- **2** CUPS LOW-SODIUM BEEF STOCK
- **2** CUPS WATER
- **2** TABLESPOON OLIVE OIL
- **½** CUP SCALLIONS, CHOPPED
- **1** CUP ARBORIO RICE
- **¼** CUP DRY WHITE WINE
- **1** CUP ROAST BEEF, THINLY STRIPPED
- **1** CUP BUTTON MUSHROOMS
- **½** CUP CANNED CREAM OF MUSHROOM
- SALT AND PEPPER AS NEEDED
- OREGANO, CHOPPED PARSLEY, CHOPPED

DIRECTION

1. Take a stock pot and put it over medium heat.
2. Add water with beef stock in it.
3. Bring the mixture to a boil and remove the heat.
4. Take another heavy-bottomed saucepan and put it over medium heat.
5. Add in the scallions and stir fry them for 1 minute.
6. Add in the rice then and cook it for at least 2 minutes, occasionally stirring it to ensure that it is finely coated with oil.

7. In the rice mixture, keep adding your beef stock ½ a cup at a time, making sure to stir it often.

8. Once all the stock has been added, cook the rice for another 2 minutes.

9. During the last 5 minutes of your cooking, make sure to add the beef, cream of mushroom, while stirring it nicely.

10. Transfer the whole mix to a serving dish.

11. Garnish with some chopped up parsley and oregano.Serve hot.

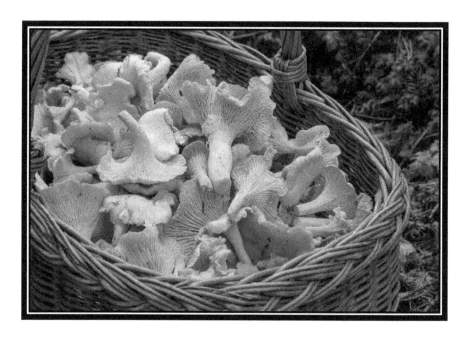

DAY 4

TUNA AND POTATOES SALAD

Preparation Time: 10 minutes
Serving: 4

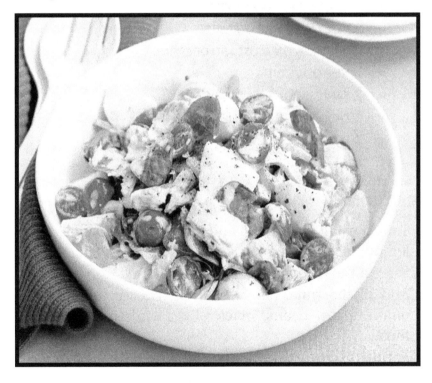

NUTRITION
Calories 406, Fat 22, Carbs 28, Protein 26

Ingredients

- 1-pound baby potatoes, scrubbed, boiled
- 1 CUP TUNA CHUNKS, DRAINED
- 1 CUP CHERRY TOMATOES, HALVED
- 1 CUP MEDIUM ONION, THINLY SLICED
- 8 PITTED BLACK OLIVES
- 2 MEDIUM HARD-BOILED EGGS, SLICED
- 1 HEAD ROMAINE LETTUCE
- HONEY LEMON MUSTARD DRESSING
- ¼ CUP OLIVE OIL
- 2 TABLESPOONS LEMON JUICE
- 1 TABLESPOON DIJON MUSTARD
- 1 TEASPOON DILL WEED, CHOPPED
- SALT AS NEEDED PEPPER AS NEEDED

Direction

1. Take a small glass bowl and mix in your olive oil, honey, lemon juice, Dijon mustard and dill.
2. Season the mix with pepper and salt.
3. Add in the tuna, baby potatoes, cherry tomatoes, red onion, green beans, black olives and toss. everything nicely.
4. Arrange your lettuce leaves on a beautiful serving dish to make the base of your salad.
5. Top them with your salad mixture and place the egg slices.
6. Drizzle it with the previously prepared Salad Dressing.
7. Serve hot.

DAY 5

BROILED MUSHROOMS BURGERS AND GOAT CHEESE

Preparation Time: 15 minutes
Cooking Time: 5 minutes
Serving: 4

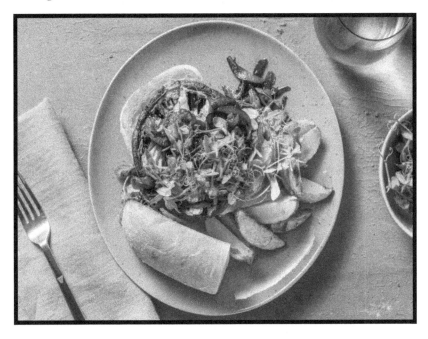

NUTRITION
Calories 327, Fat 11, Carbs 49, Protein 11

Ingredients

- **4** LARGE **P**ORTOBELLO MUSHROOM CAPS
- **1** RED ONION, CUT INTO ¼ INCH THICK SLICES
- **2** TABLESPOONS EXTRA VIRGIN OLIVE OIL
- **2** TABLESPOONS BALSAMIC VINEGAR
- PINCH OF SALT
- ¼ CUP GOAT CHEESE
- ¼ CUP SUN-DRIED TOMATOES, CHOPPED
- **4** CIABATTA BUNS **1** CUP KALE, SHREDDED

Direction

1. Pre-heat your oven to broil.
2. Take a large bowl and add mushrooms caps, onion slices, olive oil, balsamic vinegar and salt.
3. Mix well.
4. Place mushroom caps (bottom side up) and onion slices on your baking sheet.
5. Take a small bowl and stir in goat cheese and sun-dried tomatoes.
6. Toast the buns under the broiler for 30 seconds until golden.
7. Spread the goat cheese mix on top of each bun.
8. Place mushroom cap and onion slice on each bun bottom and cover with shredded kale.
9. Put everything together and serve.
10. *Enjoy!*

DAY 6

TOMATO AND HALLOUMI PLATTER

Preparation Time: 5 minutes
Cooking Time: 5 minutes
Serving: 4

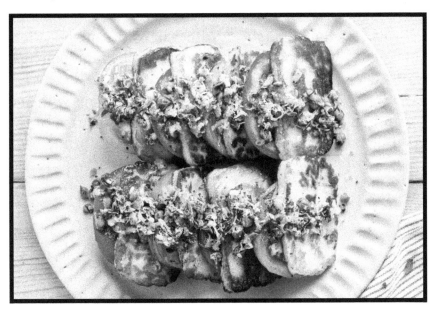

NUTRITION
Calories 109, Fat 6.7, Fiber 1.8, Carbs 1.8, Protein 9.3

Ingredients

- **1** POUND TOMATOES, SLICED
- **½** POUND HALLOUMI, CUT INTO **4** SLICES
- **2** TABLESPOONS PARSLEY, CHOPPED
- **1** TABLESPOON BASIL, CHOPPED
- **2** TABLESPOONS OLIVE OIL
- **A** PINCH OF SALT AND BLACK PEPPER JUICE OF **1** LEMON

Direction

1. Brush the halloumi slices with half of the oil, put them on your preheated grill and cook over mediumhigh heat and cook for 2 minutes on each side.
2. Arrange the tomato slices on a platter, season with salt and pepper, drizzle the lemon juice and the rest of the oil all over, top with the halloumi slices, sprinkle the herbs on top and serve for lunch.

DAY 7

Stuffed Eggplants

Preparation Time: 35 minutes
Serving: 2

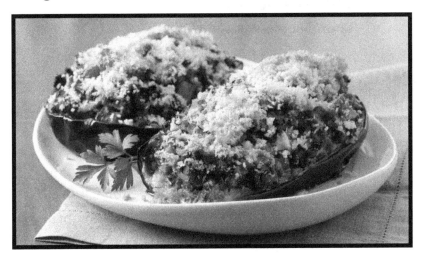

NUTRITION
Calories 512, Fat 16.4, Fiber 17.5, Carbs 78, Protein 17.2

Ingredients

- **2** EGGPLANTS, HALVED LENGTHWISE AND **2/3** OF THE FLESH SCOOPED OUT
- **3** TABLESPOONS OLIVE OIL
- **1** RED ONION, CHOPPED
- **2** GARLIC CLOVES, MINCED

- **1** PINT WHITE MUSHROOMS, SLICED
- **2** CUPS KALE, TORN
- **2** CUPS QUINOA, COOKED
- **1** TABLESPOON THYME, CHOPPED
- ZEST AND JUICE OF **1** LEMON
- SALT AND BLACK PEPPER TO THE TASTE
- ½ CUP GREEK YOGURT
- **3** TABLESPOONS PARSLEY, CHOPPED

DIRECTION

1. Rub the inside of each eggplant half with half of the oil and arrange them on a baking sheet lined with parchment paper.
2. Heat up a pan with the rest of the oil over medium heat, add the onion and the garlic and sauté for 5 minutes.
3. Add the mushrooms and cook for 5 minutes more.
4. Add the kale, salt, pepper, thyme, lemon zest and juice, stir, cook for 5 minutes more and take off the heat.
5. Stuff the eggplant halves with the mushroom mix, introduce them in the oven and bake 400 degrees F for 20 minutes.
6. Divide the eggplants between plates, sprinkle the parsley and the yogurt on top and serve for lunch.

DAY 8
SPICY POTATO SALAD

Cooking Time: 15 minutes
Serving: 4

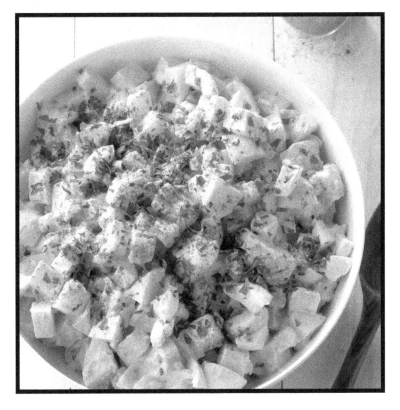

NUTRITION
Calories 354, Fat 19.2, Fiber 4.5, Carbs 24.7, Protein 11.2

INGREDIENTS

- **1 AND ½ POUNDS BABY POTATOES, PEELED AND HALVED**
- **A PINCH OF SALT AND BLACK PEPPER**
- **2 TABLESPOONS HARISSA PASTE**
- **6 OUNCES GREEK YOGURT**
- **JUICE OF 1 LEMON**
- **¼ CUP RED ONION, CHOPPED**
- **¼ CUP PARSLEY, CHOPPED**

DIRECTION

1. Put the potatoes in a pot, add water to cover, add salt, bring to a boil over medium-high heat, cook for 12 minutes, drain and transfer them to a bowl.
2. Add the harissa and the rest of the ingredients, toss and serve for lunch.

DAY 9
LENTILS SOUP

Preparation Time: 45 minutes
Servings: 6

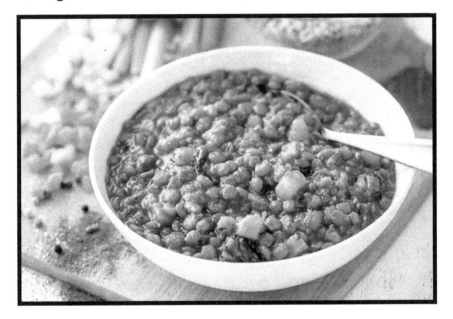

NUTRITION
Calories 238, Fat 7.3, Fiber 6.3, Carbs 32, Protein 14

Ingredients

- **1** YELLOW ONION, CHOPPED
- **2** TABLESPOONS OLIVE OIL
- **2** CELERY STALKS, CHOPPED
- **1** CARROT, SLICED
- **1/3** CUP PARSLEY, CHOPPED
- **½** CUP CILANTRO, CHOPPED
- **2 AND ½** TABLESPOONS GARLIC, MINCED
- **2** TABLESPOONS GINGER, GRATED
- **1** TEASPOON TURMERIC POWDER
- **2** TEASPOONS SWEET PAPRIKA
- **1** TEASPOON CINNAMON POWDER
- **1 AND ¼** CUPS RED LENTILS
- **15** OUNCES CANNED CHICKPEAS, DRAINED AND RINSED
- **28** OUNCES CANNED TOMATOES AND JUICE, CRUSHED
- **8** CUPS CHICKEN STOCK
- **A** PINCH OF SALT AND BLACK PEPPER

Direction

1. Heat up a pot with the oil over medium heat, add the onion, ginger, garlic, celery and carrots and sauté for 5 minutes.
2. Add the rest of the ingredients, stir, bring to a simmer over medium heat and cook for 35 minutes.
3. Ladle the soup into bowls and serve right away.

DAY 10

VEGGIE SOUP

Cooking time: 45 minutes
Servings: 8

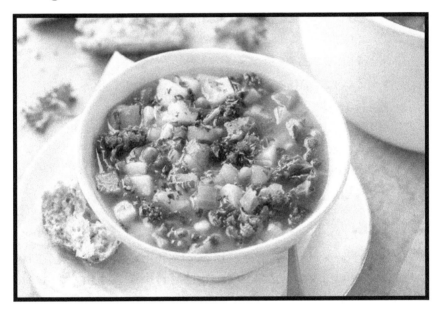

NUTRITION
Calories 300, Fat 11.3, Fiber 3.4, Carbs 17.5, Protein 10

INGREDIENTS

- **1** YELLOW ONION, CHOPPED
- **4** GARLIC CLOVES, MINCED

- ½ CUP CARROTS, CHOPPED
- 1 ZUCCHINI, CHOPPED
- 1 YELLOW SQUASH, PEELED AND CUBED
- 2 TABLESPOONS PARSLEY, CHOPPED
- 3 TABLESPOONS OLIVE OIL¼ CUP CELERY, CHOPPED
- 30 OUNCES CANNED CANNELLINI BEANS, DRAINED AND RINSED
- 30 OUNCES CANNED RED KIDNEY BEANS, DRAINED AND RINSED
- 4 CUPS VEGGIE STOCK
- 2 CUPS WATER
- ¼ TEASPOON THYME, DRIED
- ½ TEASPOON BASIL, DRIED
- A PINCH OF SALT AND BLACK PEPPER
- 4 CUPS BABY SPINACH
- ¼ CUP PARMESAN, GRATED

DIRECTION

1. Heat up a pot with the oil over medium heat, add the onion, garlic, carrots, squash, zucchini, parsley and the celery, stir and sauté for 5 minutes.
2. Add the rest of the ingredients except the spinach and the parmesan, stir, bring to a simmer over medium heat and cook for 30 minutes.
3. Add the spinach, cook the soup for 10 minutes more, divide into bowls, sprinkle the cheese on top and serve.

DAY 11
TUSCAN SOUP

Preparation Time: 15 minutes
Servings: 6

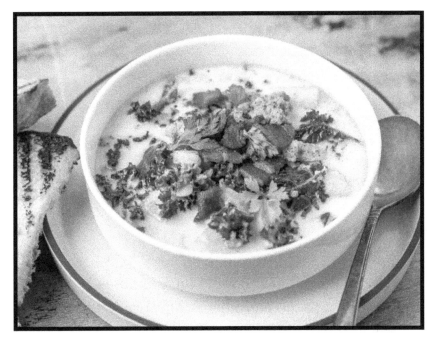

NUTRITION
Calories 471, Fat 8.2, Fiber 19.4, Carbs 76.5, Protein 27.6

INGREDIENTS

- **1** YELLOW ONION, CHOPPED
- **4** GARLIC CLOVES, MINCED
- **2** TABLESPOONS OLIVE OIL½ CUP CELERY, CHOPPED
- **½** CUP CARROTS, CHOPPED
- **15** OUNCES CANNED TOMATOES, CHOPPED
- **1** ZUCCHINI, CHOPPED
- **6** CUPS VEGGIE STOCK
- **2** TABLESPOONS TOMATO PASTE
- **15** OUNCES CANNED WHITE BEANS, DRAINED AND RINSED
- **2** HANDFULS BABY SPINACH
- **1** TABLESPOON BASIL, CHOPPED
- **SALT AND BLACK PEPPER TO THE TASTE**

DIRECTION

1. Heat up a pot with the oil over medium heat, add the garlic and the onion and sauté for 5 minutes.
2. Add the rest of the ingredients, stir, bring the soup to a simmer and cook for 10 minutes.
3. Ladle the soup into bowls and serve right away.

DAY 12

CAULIFLOWER CREAM

Preparation Time: 1h 10 minutes
Servings: 8

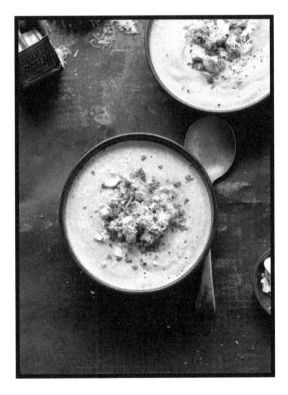

NUTRITION
Calories 243, Fat 17, Fiber 2.3, Carbs 41.1, Protein 13.7

INGREDIENTS

- **1** CAULIFLOWER HEAD, FLORETS SEPARATED
- **1** TEASPOON GARLIC POWDER
- **2** TABLESPOONS OLIVE OIL
- **1** YELLOW ONION, CHOPPED
- SALT AND BLACK PEPPER TO THE TASTE
- **5** CUPS CHICKEN STOCK
- **2** TABLESPOONS GARLIC, MINCED
- **2** AND ½ CUPS CHEDDAR CHEESE, SHREDDED

DIRECTION

1. Spread the cauliflower on a baking sheet lined with parchment paper, add garlic powder, half of the oil, salt and pepper and roast at 425 degrees F for 30 minutes.
2. Heat up a pot with the rest of the oil over medium heat, add the onion and sauté for 5 minutes.
3. Add the roasted cauliflower and the rest of the ingredients except the cheddar, stir and simmer the soup for 30 minutes.
4. Blend the soup using an immersion blender, add the cheese, stir, divide the soup into bowls and serve.

DAY 13

BASIL ZUCCHINI SOUP

Preparation Time: 20 minutes
Servings: 4

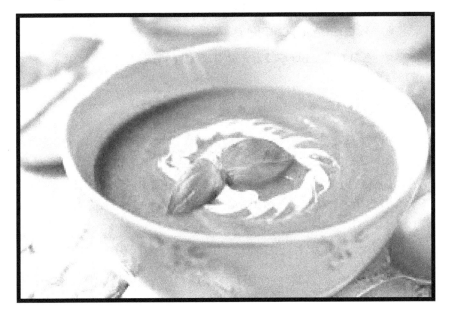

NUTRITION
Calories 274, Fat 11.2, Fiber 4.5, Carbs 16.5, Protein 4.5

INGREDIENTS

- **2** TABLESPOONS OLIVE OIL
- **3** GARLIC CLOVES, MINCED
- **1** YELLOW ONION, CHOPPED
- **4** ZUCCHINIS, CUBED
- **4** CUPS CHICKEN STOCK
- ZEST OF **1** LEMON, GRATED
- ½ CUP BASIL, CHOPPED
- SALT AND BLACK PEPPER TO THE TASTE

DIRECTION

1. Heat up a pot with the oil over medium heat, add the onion and the garlic and sauté for 5 minutes.
2. Add the zucchinis and the rest of the ingredients except the basil, bring to a simmer and cook over medium heat for 15 minutes.
3. Add the basil, stir, and divide the soup into bowls and serve.

DAY 14

WHITE BEANS AND ORANGE SOUP

Preparation Time: 37 minutes
Servings: 4

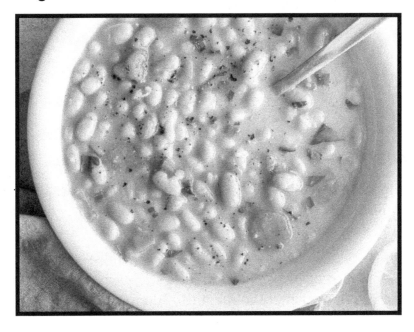

NUTRITION
Calories 273, Fat 16.3, Fiber 8.4, Carbs 15.6, Protein 7.4

INGREDIENTS

- **1** YELLOW ONION, CHOPPED
- **5** CELERY STICKS, CHOPPED
- **4** CARROTS, CHOPPED
- **1** CUP OLIVE OIL
- **½** TEASPOON OREGANO, DRIED
- **1** BAY LEAF
- **3** ORANGE SLICES, PEELED
- **30** OUNCES CANNED WHITE BEANS, DRAINED
- **2** TABLESPOONS TOMATO PASTE
- **2** CUPS WATER
- **6** CUPS CHICKEN STOCK

DIRECTION

1. Heat up a pot with the oil over medium heat, add the onion, celery, carrots, the bay leaf and the oregano, stir and sauté for 5 minutes.
2. Add the orange slices and cook for 2 minutes more.
3. Add the rest of the ingredients, stir, bring to a simmer and cook over medium heat for 30 minutes.
4. Ladle the soup into bowls and serve.

Chapter 2

14 DAYS – DINNERS

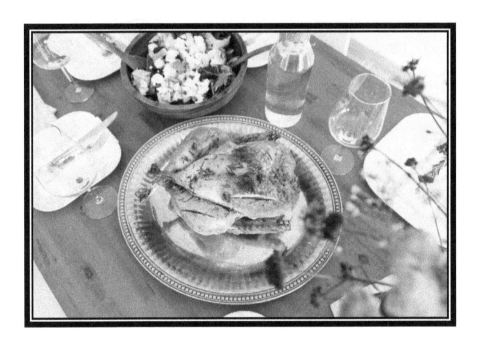

DAY 01

MEDITERRANEAN LAMB CHOPS

Preparation Time: 10 minutes
Cooking Time: 10 minutes
Serving: 4

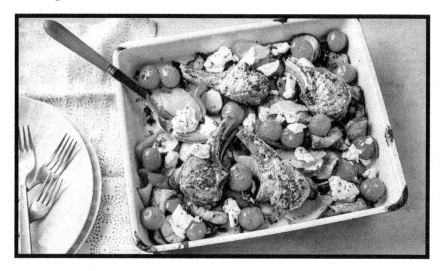

NUTRITION
Calories: 521, Fat: 45g, Carbohydrates: 3.5g, Protein: 22g

INGREDIENTS

- 4 LAMB SHOULDER CHOPS, 8 OUNCE EACH
- 2 TABLESPOONS DIJON MUSTARD

- **2** TABLESPOONS **B**ALSAMIC VINEGAR
- **1** TABLESPOON GARLIC, CHOPPED
- ½ CUP OLIVE OIL
- **2** TABLESPOONS SHREDDED FRESH BASIL

DIRECTION

1. Pat your lamb chop dry using kitchen towel and arrange them on a shallow glass baking dish.
2. Take a bowl and whisk in Dijon mustard, balsamic vinegar, garlic, pepper and mix well.
3. Whisk in the oil very slowly into the marinade until the mixture is smooth.
4. Stir in basil.
5. Pour the marinade over the lamb chops and stir to coat both sides well.
6. Cover the chops and allow them to marinate for 1-4 hours (chilled).
7. Take the chops out and leave them for 30 minutes to allow the temperature to reach normal level.
8. Pre-heat your grill to medium heat and add oil to the grate.
9. Grill the lamb chops for 5-10 minutes per side until both sides are browned.
10. Once the center of the chop reads 145-degree Fahrenheit, the chops are ready, serve and enjoy!

DAY 02

MUSHROOM AND PORK CHOPS

Preparation Time: 10 minutes
Cooking Time: 25 minutes
Serving: 4

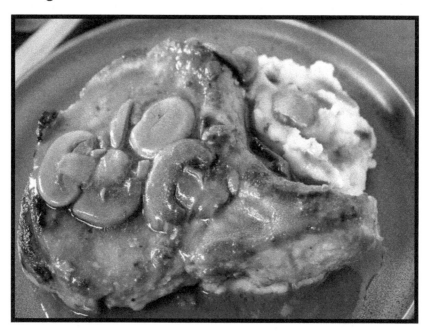

NUTRITION
Calories: 308, Fat: 17g, Carbohydrates: 7g, Protein 33

INGREDIENTS

- **4 (5 OUNCE) BONE-IN-CENTER PORK CHOPS**
- **¼ TEASPOON SEA SALT**
- **¼ TEASPOON FRESHLY GROUND BLACK PEPPER**
- **1 TABLESPOON EXTRA-VIRGIN OLIVE OIL**
- **1 SWEET ONION, CHOPPED**
- **2 TEASPOONS GARLIC, MINCED**
- **1-POUND MIXED WILD MUSHROOMS, SLICED**
- **1 TEASPOON FRESH THYME, CHOPPED ½ CUP SODIUM FREE CHICKEN STOCK**

DIRECTION

1. Pat pork chops dry with kitchen towel and season with salt and pepper.
2. Take a large skillet and place it over medium-high heat.
3. Add olive oil and heat it up.
4. Add pork chops and cook for 6 minutes, brown both sides.
5. Transfer meat to platter and keep it aside.
6. Add onion and garlic and sauté for 3 minutes.
7. Stir in mushrooms and thyme and sauté for 6 minutes until the mushrooms are caramelized.
8. Return pork chops to the skillet and pour chicken stock.
9. Cover and bring liquid to boil.
10. Reduce the heat to low and simmer for 10 minutes.
11. Serve and Enjoy.

DAY 03

CHICKEN SKILLET

Preparation Time: 35 minutes
Serving: 6

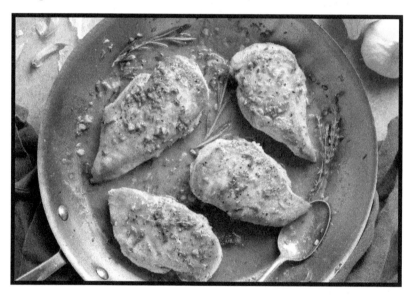

NUTRITION
Calories: 435, Fat: 18.5g, Fiber 13.6, Carbohydrates: 27.8g,
Protein: 25.6g

INGREDIENTS

- 6 CHICKEN THIGHS, BONE-IN AND SKIN-ON
- JUICE OF 2 LEMONS

- **1** TEASPOON OREGANO, DRIED
- **1** RED ONION, CHOPPED
- SALT AND BLACK PEPPER TO THE TASTE
- **1** TEASPOON GARLIC POWDER
- **2** GARLIC CLOVES, MINCED
- **2** TABLESPOONS OLIVE OIL
- **2** AND ½ CUPS CHICKEN STOCK
- **1** CUP WHITE RICE
- **1** TABLESPOON OREGANO, CHOPPED
- **1** CUP GREEN OLIVES, PITTED AND SLICED
- **1/3** CUP PARSLEY, CHOPPED
- ½ CUP FETA CHEESE, CRUMBLED

DIRECTION

1. Heat up a pan with the oil over medium heat, add the chicken thighs skin side down, cook for 4 minutes on each side and transfer to a plate.
2. Add the garlic and the onion to the pan, stir and sauté for 5 minutes.
3. Add the rice, salt, pepper, the stock, oregano, and lemon juice, stir, cook for 1-2 minutes more and take off the heat.
4. Add the chicken to the pan, introduce the pan in the oven and bake at 375 degrees F for 25 minutes.
5. Add the cheese, olives and the parsley, divide the whole mix between plates and serve for dinner.

DAY 04

TUNA AND COUSCOUS

Preparation Time: 10 minutes
Serving: 4

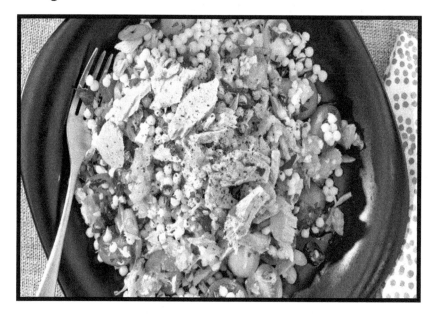

NUTRITION
Calories: 253, Fat: 11.5g, Fiber 3.4, Carbohydrates: 16.5g,
Protein: 23.2g

INGREDIENTS

- **1** CUP CHICKEN STOCK
- **1** AND ¼ CUPS COUSCOUS
- **A** PINCH OF SALT AND BLACK PEPPER
- **10** OUNCES CANNED TUNA, DRAINED AND FLAKED
- **1** PINT CHERRY TOMATOES, HALVED
- **½** CUP PEPPERONCINI, SLICED
- **1/3** CUP PARSLEY, CHOPPED
- **1** TABLESPOON OLIVE OIL
- **¼** CUP CAPERS, DRAINED JUICE OF ½ LEMON

DIRECTION

1. Put the stock in a pan, bring to a boil over medium-high heat, add the couscous, stir, take off the heat, cover, leave aside for 10 minutes, fluff with a fork and transfer to a bowl.
2. Add the tuna and the rest of the ingredients, toss and serve for dinner right away.

DAY 05

TURKEY FRITTERS AND SAUCE

Preparation Time: 30 minutes
Serving: 2

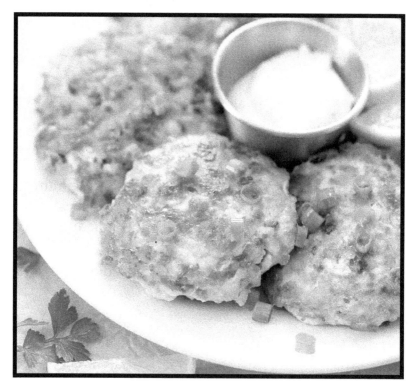

NUTRITION
Calories: 364 Fat: 16.8g, Fiber 5.5, Carbohydrates: 26.8g, Protein: 23.4g

---

INGREDIENTS

- **2** GARLIC CLOVES, MINCED
- **1** EGG
- **1** RED ONION, CHOPPED
- **1** TABLESPOON OLIVE OIL
- **¼** TEASPOON RED PEPPER FLAKES
- **1** POUND TURKEY MEAT, GROUND
- **½** TEASPOON OREGANO, DRIED COOKING SPRAY

FOR THE SAUCE:

- **1** CUP GREEK YOGURT
- **1** CUCUMBER, CHOPPED
- **1** TABLESPOON OLIVE OIL
- **¼** TEASPOON GARLIC POWDER
- **2** TABLESPOONS LEMON JUICE
- **¼** CUP PARSLEY, CHOPPED

DIRECTION

1. Heat up a pan with 1 tablespoon oil over medium heat, add the onion and the garlic, sauté for 5 minutes, cool down and transfer to a bowl.
2. Add the meat, turkey, oregano and pepper flakes, stir and shape medium fritters out of this mix.

---

3. Heat up another pan greased with cooking spray over medium-high heat, add the turkey fritters and brown for 5 minutes on each side.

4. Introduce the pan in the oven and bake the fritters at 375 degrees F for 15 minutes more.

5. Meanwhile, in a bowl, mix the yogurt with the cucumber, oil, garlic powder, lemon juice and parsley and whisk really well.

6. Divide the fritters between plates, spread the sauce all over and serve for dinner.

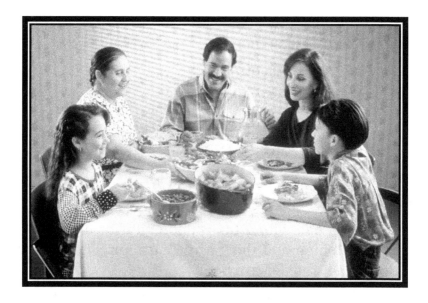

DAY 06

SALMON BOWL

Preparation Time: 40 minutes
Serving: 4

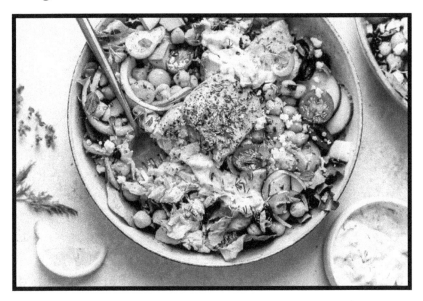

NUTRITION

Calories: 281, Carbohydrates: 5.8g, Fat: 12.7g, Protein 36.5, Fiber
1.7

INGREDIENTS

- **2** CUPS FARRO
- JUICE OF **2** LEMONS

85

- **1/3** CUP OLIVE OIL+ **2** TABLESPOONS
- **SALT AND BLACK PEPPER**
- **1** CUCUMBER, CHOPPED
- **¼** CUP BALSAMIC VINEGAR
- **1** GARLIC CLOVES, MINCED
- **¼** CUP PARSLEY, CHOPPED
- **¼** CUP MINT, CHOPPED
- **2** TABLESPOONS MUSTARD
- **4** SALMON FILLETS, BONELESS

DIRECTION

1. Put water in a large pot, bring to a boil over medium-high heat, add salt and the farro, stir, simmer for 30 minutes, drain, transfer to a bowl, add the lemon juice, mustard, garlic, salt, pepper and 1/3 cup oil, toss and leave aside for now.
2. In another bowl, mash the cucumber with a fork, add the vinegar, salt, pepper, the parsley, dill and mint and whisk well.
3. Heat up a pan with the rest of the oil over medium heat, add the salmon fillets skin side down, cook for 5 minutes on each side, cool them down and break into pieces.
4. Add over the farro, add the cucumber dressing, toss and serve for dinner.

DAY 07

SEAFOOD GUMBO

Preparation Time: 30 minutes

Servings: 4

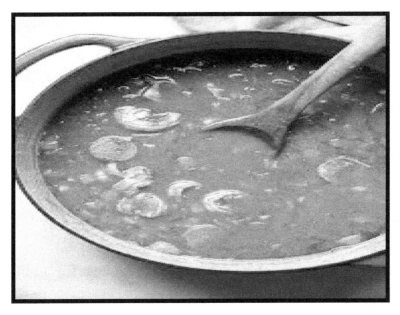

NUTRITION

Calories 363, Fat 2, Fiber 5, Carbs 18, Protein 40

INGREDIENTS

- ¼ CUP TAPIOCA FLOUR
- ¼ CUP OLIVE OIL

- **1** CUP CELERY, CHOPPED
- **1** WHITE ONION, CHOPPED
- **1** RED BELL PEPPER, CHOPPED
- **1** GREEN BELL PEPPER, CHOPPED
- **1** RED CHILI, CHOPPED
- **2** CUPS OKRA, CHOPPED
- **2** GARLIC CLOVES, MINCED
- **1** CUP CANNED TOMATOES, CRUSHED
- **1** TEASPOON THYME, DRIED
- **2** CUPS FISH STOCK
- **1** BAY LEAF
- **16** OUNCES CANNED CRAB MEAT, DRAINED
- **1** POUND SHRIMP, PEELED AND DEVEINED
- **¼** CUP PARSLEY, CHOPPED
- SALT AND BLACK PEPPER TO THE TASTE

DIRECTION

1. Heat up a pot with the oil over medium heat, add the flour, whisk to obtain a paste and cook for about 5 minutes.
2. Add the bell peppers, the onions, celery and the okra and sauté for 5 minutes.
3. Add the rest of the ingredients except the crab, shrimp, and parsley, stir, bring to a simmer and cook for 15 minutes.
4. Add the remaining ingredients, simmer the soup for 10 minutes more, divide into bowls and serve.

DAY 08

FISH AND TOMATO SAUCE

Preparation Time: 10 minutes
Cooking Time: 30 minutes
Servings: 4

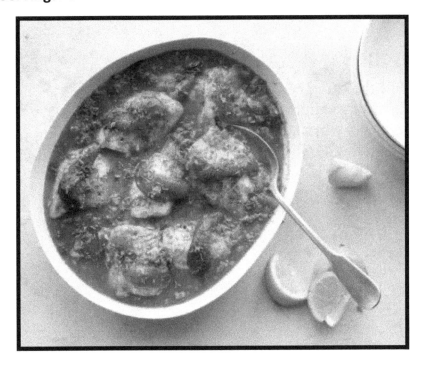

NUTRITION
Calories 180, Fat 23, Fiber 12, Carbs 23, Protein 25

INGREDIENTS

- **4** COD FILLETS, BONELESS
- **2** GARLIC CLOVES, MINCED
- **2** CUPS CHERRY TOMATOES, HALVED
- **1** CUP CHICKEN STOCK
- **A** PINCH OF SALT AND BLACK PEPPER
- **¼** CUP BASIL, CHOPPED

DIRECTION

1. Put the tomatoes, garlic, salt and pepper in a pan, heat up over medium heat and cook for 5 minutes.
2. Add the fish and the rest of the ingredients, bring to a simmer, cover the pan and cook for 25 minutes. Divide the mix between plates and serve.

DAY 09

LEMON AND DATES BARRAMUNDI

Preparation Time: 10 minutes
Cooking Time: 12 minutes
Servings: 2

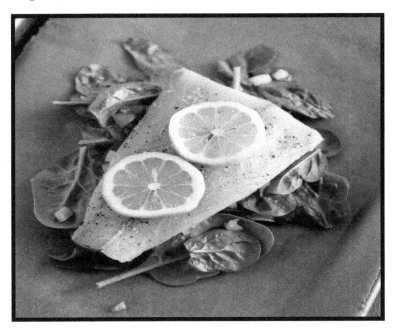

NUTRITION
Calories 232, Fat 23, Fiber 12, Carbs 23, Protein 25

Ingredients

- **2** BARRAMUNDI FILLETS, BONELESS
- **1** SHALLOT, SLICED
- **4** LEMON SLICES
- JUICE OF ½ LEMON
- ZEST OF **1** LEMON, GRATED
- **2** TABLESPOONS OLIVE OIL
- **6** OUNCES BABY SPINACH
- ¼ CUP ALMONDS, CHOPPED
- **4** DATES, PITTED AND CHOPPED
- ¼ CUP PARSLEY, CHOPPED
- SALT AND BLACK PEPPER TO THE TASTE

Direction

1. Season the fish with salt and pepper and arrange on 2 parchment paper pieces.
2. Top the fish with the lemon slices, drizzle the lemon juice, and then top with the other DAY 10

DAY 10

FISH CAKE

Preparation Time: 10 minutes
Cooking Time: 10 minutes
Servings: 6

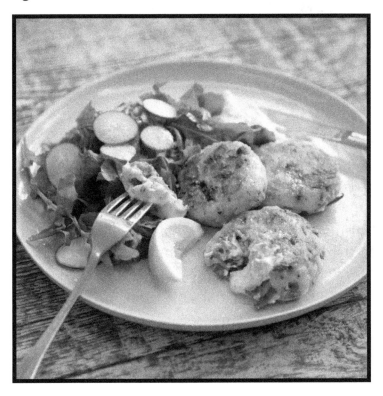

NUTRITION
Calories 402, Fat 23, Fiber 12, Carbs 23, Protein 25

INGREDIENTS

- **20** OUNCES CANNED SARDINES, DRAINED AND MASHED WELL
- **2** GARLIC CLOVES, MINCED
- **2** TABLESPOONS DILL, CHOPPED
- **1** YELLOW ONION, CHOPPED
- **1** CUP PANKO BREADCRUMBS
- **1** EGG, WHISKED
- **A** PINCH OF SALT AND BLACK PEPPER
- **2** TABLESPOONS LEMON JUICE
- **5** TABLESPOONS OLIVE OIL

DIRECTION

1. In a bowl, combine the sardines with the garlic, dill and the rest of the ingredients except the oil, stir well and shape medium cakes out of this mix.
2. Heat up a pan with the oil over medium-high heat, add the fish cakes, cook for 5 minutes on each side. Serve the cakes with a side salad.

DAY 11

DUCK, CUCUMBER AND MANGO SALAD

Preparation Time: 50 minutes
Servings: 4

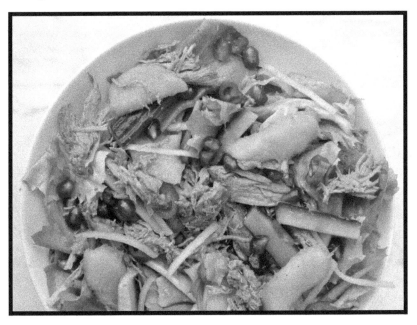

NUTRITION
Calories 297, Fat 9.1, Fiber 10,2, Carbs 20.8, Protein 16.5

INGREDIENTS

- ZEST OF 1 ORANGE, GRATED
- 2 BIG DUCK BREASTS, BONELESS AND SKIN SCORED
- 2 TABLESPOONS OLIVE OIL
- SALT AND BLACK PEPPER TO THE TASTE
- 1 TABLESPOON FISH SAUCE 1 TABLESPOON LIME JUICE
- 1 GARLIC CLOVE, MINCED
- 1 SERRANO CHILI, CHOPPED
- 1 SMALL SHALLOT, SLICED
- 1 CUCUMBER, SLICED
- 2 MANGOS, PEELED AND SLICED
- ¼ CUP OREGANO, CHOPPED

DIRECTION

1. Heat up a pan with the oil over medium-high heat, add the duck breasts skin side down and cook for 5 minutes.
2. Add the orange zest, salt, pepper, fish sauce and the rest of the ingredients, bring to a simmer and cook over medium-low heat for 45 minutes.
3. Divide everything between plates and serve.

DAY 12

GLAZED PORK CHOPS

Preparation Time: 20 minutes
Servings: 4

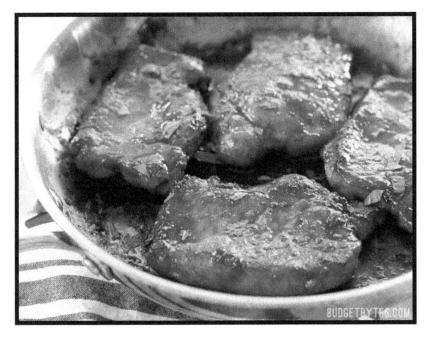

NUTRITION
Calories 225, Fat 11, Carbs 6, Protein 23

INGREDIENTS

- ¼ CUP APRICOT PRESERVES
- 4 PORK CHOPS, BONELESS
- 1 TABLESPOON THYME, CHOPPED
- ½ TEASPOON CINNAMON POWDER
- 2 TABLESPOONS OLIVE OIL

DIRECTION

1. Heat up a pan with the oil over medium-high heat, add the apricot preserves and cinnamon, whisk, bring to a simmer, cook for 10 minutes and take off the heat.
2. Heat up your grill over medium-high heat, brush the pork chops with some of the apricot glaze, place them on the grill and cook for 10 minutes.
3. Flip the chops, brush them with more apricot glaze, cook for 10 minutes more and divide between plates.
4. Sprinkle the thyme on top and serve.

DAY 13
HALIBUT PAN

Preparation 10 minutes
Cooking Time: 20 minutes
Servings: 4

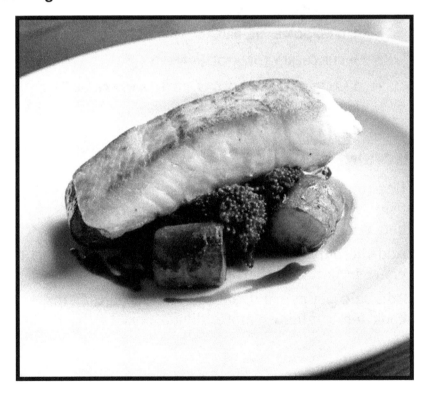

NUTRITION
Calories 402, Fat 23, Fiber 12, Carbs 23, Protein 25

INGREDIENTS

- **4** HALIBUT FILLETS, BONELESS
- **1** RED BELL PEPPER, CHOPPED
- **2** TABLESPOONS OLIVE OIL
- **1** YELLOW ONION, CHOPPED
- **4** GARLIC CLOVES, MINCED
- **½** CUP CHICKEN STOCK
- **1** TEASPOON BASIL, DRIED
- **½** CUP CHERRY TOMATOES, HALVED
- **1/3** CUP KALAMATA OLIVES, PITTED AND HALVED SALT AND BLACK PEPPER TO THE TASTE

DIRECTION

1. Heat up a pan with the oil over medium heat, add the fish, cook for 5 minutes on each side and divide between plates.
2. Add the onion, bell pepper, garlic and tomatoes to the pan, stir and sauté for 3 minutes.
3. Add salt, pepper and the rest of the ingredients, toss, cook for 3 minutes more, divide next to the fish and serve.

DAY 14

BAKED SHRIMP MIX

Preparation Time: 10 minutes
Cooking Time: 32 minutes
Servings: 4

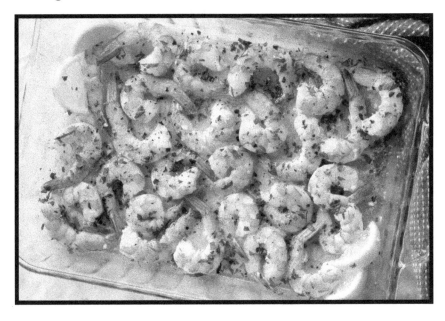

NUTRITION
Calories 341, Fat 23, Fiber 12, Carbs 23, Protein 25

INGREDIENTS

- **4** GOLD POTATOES, PEELED AND SLICED
- **2** FENNEL BULBS, TRIMMED AND CUT INTO WEDGES
- **2** SHALLOTS, CHOPPED
- **2** GARLIC CLOVES, MINCED
- **3** TABLESPOONS OLIVE OIL
- **½** CUP KALAMATA OLIVES, PITTED AND HALVED
- **2** POUNDS SHRIMP, PEELED AND DEVEINED
- **1** TEASPOON LEMON ZEST, GRATED
- **2** TEASPOONS OREGANO, DRIED
- **4** OUNCES FETA CHEESE, CRUMBLED
- **2** TABLESPOONS PARSLEY, CHOPPED

DIRECTION

1. In a roasting pan, combine the potatoes with 2 tablespoons oil, garlic and the rest of the ingredients except the shrimp, toss, introduce in the oven and bake at 450 degrees F for 25 minutes.
2. Add the shrimp, toss, bake for 7 minutes more, divide between plates and serve.

Chapter 3

EXTRA ENERGY-DESSERTS

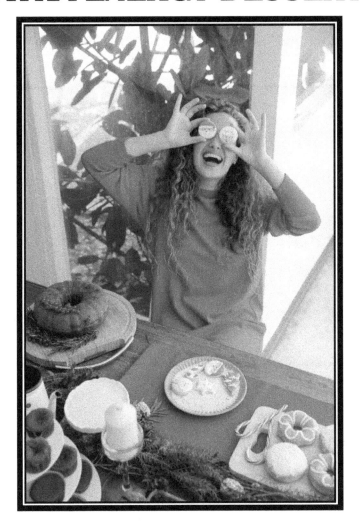

01
COLD LEMON SQUARES

Preparation time: 30 minutes
Servings: 4

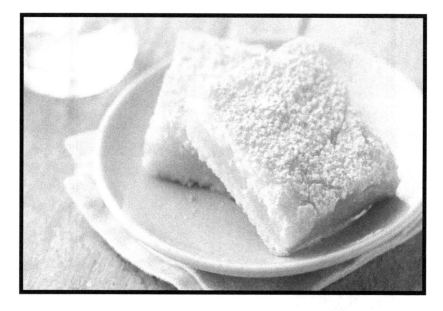

NUTRITION
Calories 136, Fat 11.2, Fiber 0.2, Carbs 7, Protein 1.1

Ingredients

- **1** CUP AVOCADO OIL+ A DRIZZLE
- **2** BANANAS, PEELED AND CHOPPED
- **1** TABLESPOON HONEY
- **¼** CUP LEMON JUICE
- **A** PINCH OF LEMON ZEST, GRATED

Direction

1. In your food processor, mix the bananas with the rest of the ingredients, pulse well and spread on the bottom of a pan greased with a drizzle of oil.
2. Introduce in the fridge for 30 minutes, slice into squares and serve.

02

GREEN TEA AND VANILLA CREAM

Preparation time: 2h
Servings: 4

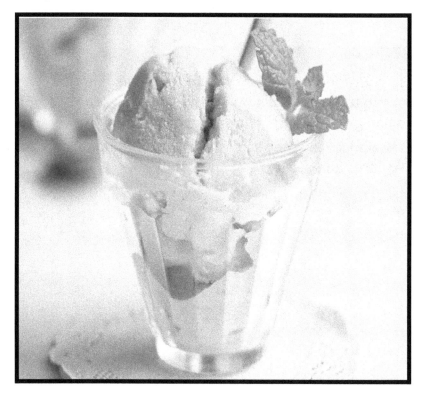

NUTRITION
Calories 120, Fat 3, Fiber 3, Carbs 7, Protein 4

INGREDIENTS

- **14** OUNCES ALMOND MILK, HOT
- **2** TABLESPOONS GREEN TEA POWDER
- **14** OUNCES HEAVY CREAM
- **3** TABLESPOONS STEVIA
- **1** TEASPOON VANILLA EXTRACT
- **1** TEASPOON GELATIN POWDER

DIRECTION

1. In a bowl, combine the almond milk with the green tea powder and the rest of the ingredients, whisk well, cool down, divide into cups and keep in the fridge for 2 hours before serving.

03

PEACH SORBET

Preparation time: 2h
Servings: 4

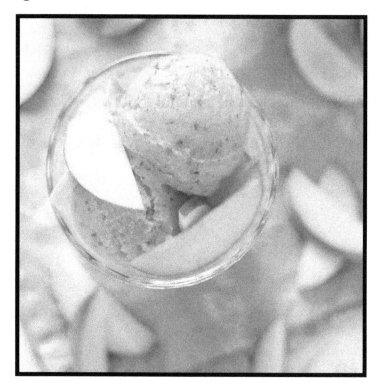

NUTRITION
Calories 182, Fat 5.4, Fiber 3.4, Carbs 12, Protein 5.4

INGREDIENTS

- **2** CUPS APPLE JUICE
- **1** CUP STEVIA
- **2** TABLESPOONS LEMON ZEST, GRATED
- **2** POUNDS PEACHES, PITTED AND qUARTERED

DIRECTION

1. Heat up a pan over medium heat, add the apple juice and the rest of the ingredients, simmer for 10 minutes, transfer to a blender, pulse, divide into cups and keep in the freezer for 2 hours before serving.

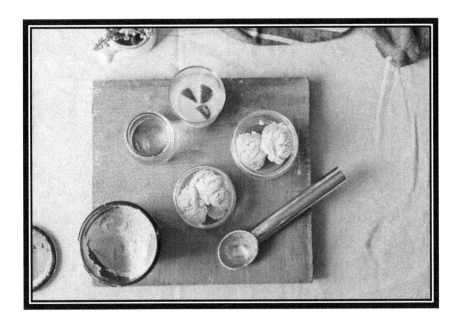

04

LEMON CREAM

Preparation time: 1h
Servings: 6

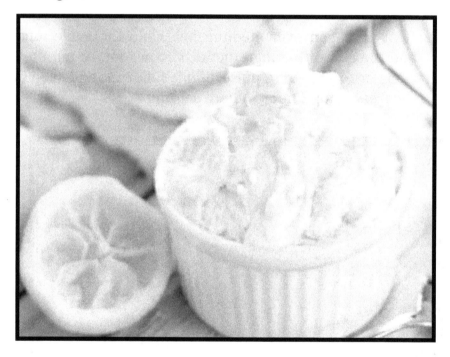

NUTRITION
Calories 200, Fat 8.5, Fiber 4.5, Carbs 8.6, Protein 4.5

INGREDIENTS

- **2** EGGS, WHISKED
- **1** AND **¼** CUP STEVIA
- **10** TABLESPOONS AVOCADO OIL
- **1** CUP HEAVY CREAM
- JUICE OF **2** LEMONS
- ZEST OF **2** LEMONS, GRATED

DIRECTION

1. In a pan, combine the cream with the lemon juice and the other ingredients, whisk well, cook for 10 minutes, divide into cups and keep in the fridge for 1 hour before serving.

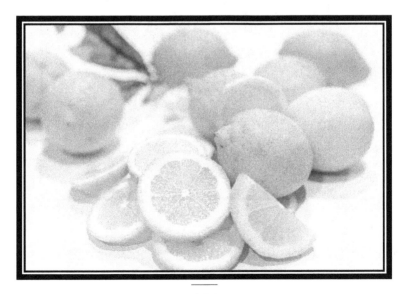

05

BLUEBERRY STEWED

Preparation time: 10 minutes
Servings: 4

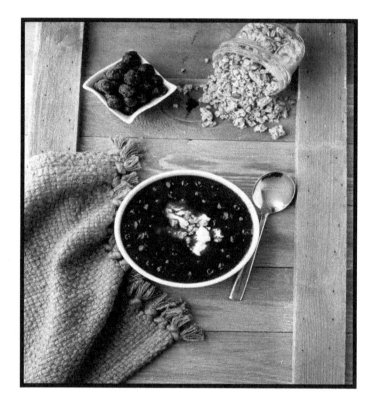

NUTRITION
Calories 192, Fat 5.4, Fiber 3.4, Carbs 9.4, Protein 4.5

INGREDIENTS

- **2** CUPS BLUEBERRIES
- **3** TABLESPOONS STEVIA
- **1** AND ½ CUPS PURE APPLE JUICE
- **1** TEASPOON VANILLA EXTRACT

DIRECTION

1. In a pan, combine the blueberries with stevia and the other ingredients, bring to a simmer and cook over medium-low heat for 10 minutes.
2. Divide into cups and serve cold.

06

MANDARIN CREAM

Preparation time: 20 minutes
Servings: 8

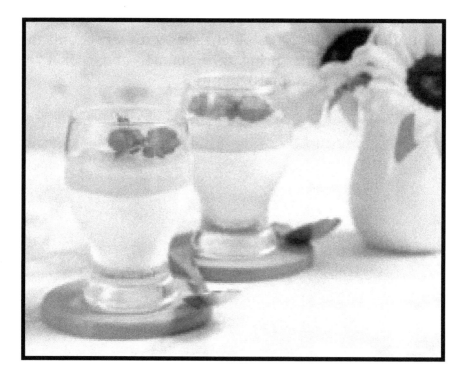

NUTRITION
Calories 106, Fat 3.4,, Carbs 2.4, Protein 4

INGREDIENTS

- **2** MANDARINS, PEELED AND CUT INTO SEGMENTS
- JUICE OF **2** MANDARINS
- **2** TABLESPOONS STEVIA
- **4** EGGS, WHISKED
- ¾ CUP STEVIA
- ¾ CUP ALMONDS, GROUND

DIRECTION

1. In a blender, combine the mandarins with the mandarins juice and the other ingredients, whisk well, divide into cups and keep in the fridge for 20 minutes before serving.

07

Cocoa and Pears Cream

Preparation time: 10 minutes
Servings: 4

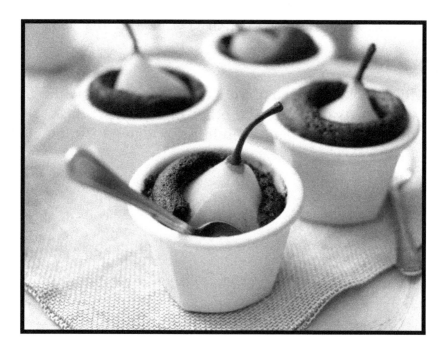

NUTRITION
Calories 172, Fat 5.6, Fiber 3.5, Carbs 7.6, Protein 4

INGREDIENTS

- **2** CUPS HEAVY CREAMY
- **1/3** CUP STEVIA
- **¾** CUP COCOA POWDER
- **6** OUNCES DARK CHOCOLATE, CHOPPED
- ZEST OF **1** LEMON
- **2** PEARS, CHOPPED

DIRECTION

1. In a blender, combine the cream with the stevia and the rest of the ingredients, pulse well, divide into cups and serve cold.

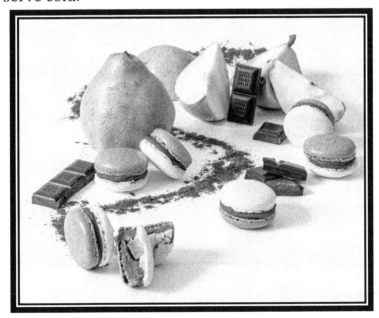

08

CREAMY MINT STRAWBERRY MIX

Preparation time: 30 minutes
Servings: 6

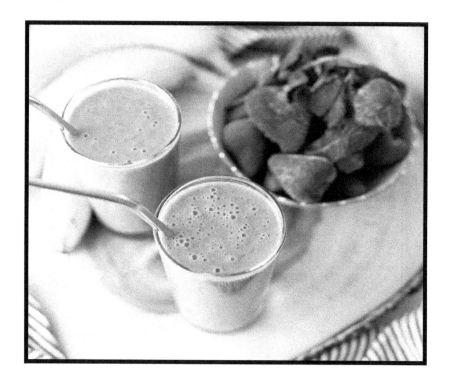

NUTRITION
Calories 200, Fat 6.3, Fiber 2, Carbs 6.5, Protein 8

INGREDIENTS

- COOKING SPRAY
- ¼ CUP STEVIA
- 1 AND ½ CUP ALMOND FLOUR
- 1 TEASPOON BAKING POWDER
- 1 CUP ALMOND MILK
- 1 EGG, WHISKED
- 2 CUPS STRAWBERRIES, SLICED
- 1 TABLESPOON MINT, CHOPPED
- 1 TEASPOON LIME ZEST, GRATED
- ½ CUP WHIPPING CREAM

DIRECTION

1. In a bowl, combine the almond with the strawberries, mint and the other ingredients except the cooking spray and whisk well.
2. Grease 6 ramekins with the cooking spray, pour the strawberry mix inside, introduce in the oven and bake at 350 degrees F for 30 minutes.
3. Cool down and serve.

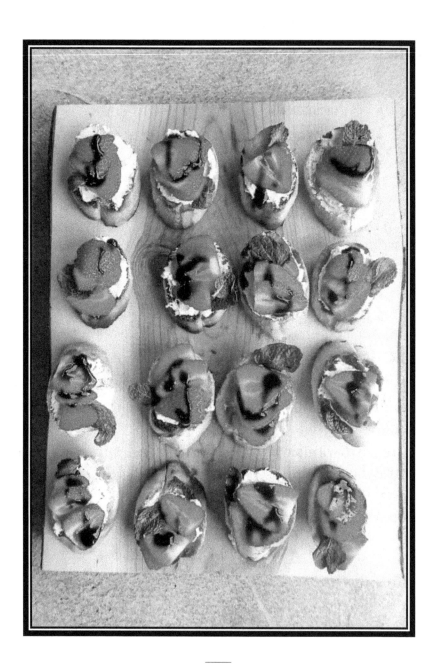

CONCLUSION

A WORD ABOUT EXTREME CALORIE RESTRICTION

Unfortunately, it is not uncommon to see some diets recommend extremely low calorie goals, such as below 1,200 calories. These levels are unlikely to sustain the energy needs of most healthy people for any length of time.

Additionally, along with the calorie restriction and unmet nutritional needs comes the question of the impact such restriction has on your metabolism. "When we go for long periods without food, our body starts to conserve energy, as it doesn't know when the next meal is coming," Andrews explains. "In basic terms, your body is going to lose water weight first, followed by some muscle tissue, and then it is going to slow down your metabolism and conserve fat as a consequence."

Extreme calorie restriction, as well as excessive exercising without adequate calorie intake, can have lasting consequences on health, as Andrews explains. "While you may see some immediate movement on the scale, this won't equate to long-term results once you start eating normally again," she says. "And it could take time for your metabolism to recover. In addition, if your diet isn't meeting your micronutrient needs, you could see systemic effects, from brittle nails to hair breakage and impaired immunity." Other lasting consequences, such as amenorrhea (absence of menstruation) and decreased bone density, may also result from consuming inadequate calories over a long period of time.

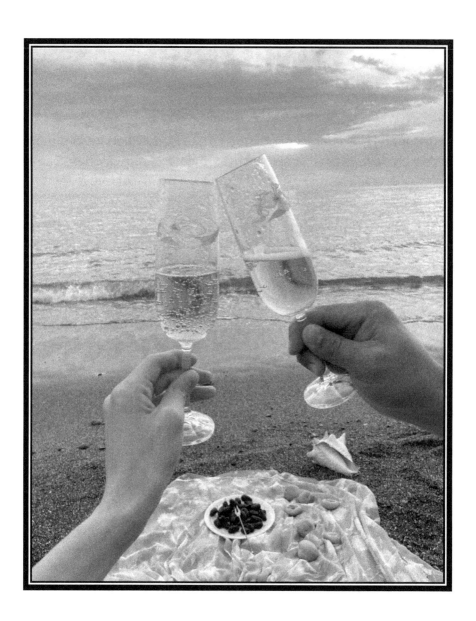

THANK YOU

FOR CHOOSING MY BOOK

AND TRYING OUT

MY DELICIOUS MEDITERRANEAN RECIPES!

ABOUT MARGARET RALLS

Margaret Ralls is a proficient chef and dietitian and has experience of over 15 years.

She is also the owner of some farmhouse that she has started in Italy, in Brittany but also in South England.

Margaret likes to travel to different countries and organize meetings for beginners to share her experience and some secret to make inexpressible and tasty dishes.

Many of these recipes you can see in the cookbooks that the author creates with love.
If you have refined taste and don't want to waste your time, just make your life easier and healthier with the recipes that advise Margaret.

.

CPSIA information can be obtained
at www.ICGtesting.com
Printed in the USA
BVHW041526210521
607795BV00001B/377